SIMPLY SMART
SUPPER SALADS
COOKBOOK

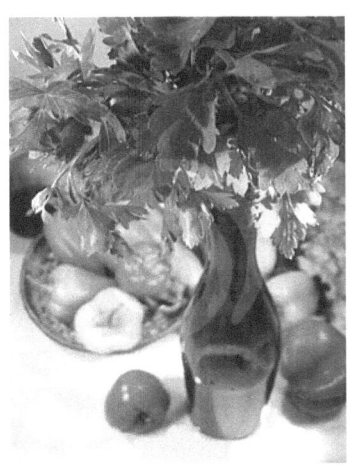

By: Lawander D. Harris

IN THE LIGHT OF HIS WORD MINISTRY

COPYRIGHT PAGE

TABLE OF CONTENTS

(1) BOWTYE PASTA SUPPER SALAD

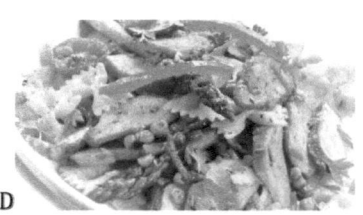

Ingredients

* 2 ½ cups uncooked bow tie pasta

* 1 cup of fresh asparagus

*1 ½ cups cubed cooked chicken breast

*1 medium tomato, diced

* 4 bacon strips, cooked and crumbled

* 1/3 cup reduced-fat salad dressing

*1/4 cup water (to boil pasta)

*1/4 teaspoon pepper

*1/4 teaspoon sea salt

* 1/4 teaspoon chili & dill seasoning

*1/2 cup green sweet peas

*1/4 cup Zucchini

* 1/3 cup of red bell pepper strips

Directions

Cook pasta according to package directions. Drain and rinse under cold water. In a large serving bowl, combine the pasta, asparagus, chicken, tomato, sweet peas, zucchini, bells and bacon. In a small bowl, whisk together the fat free dressing with dry seasonings, Pour over pasta mixture; toss to coat evenly. Serve with yummy pleasure!

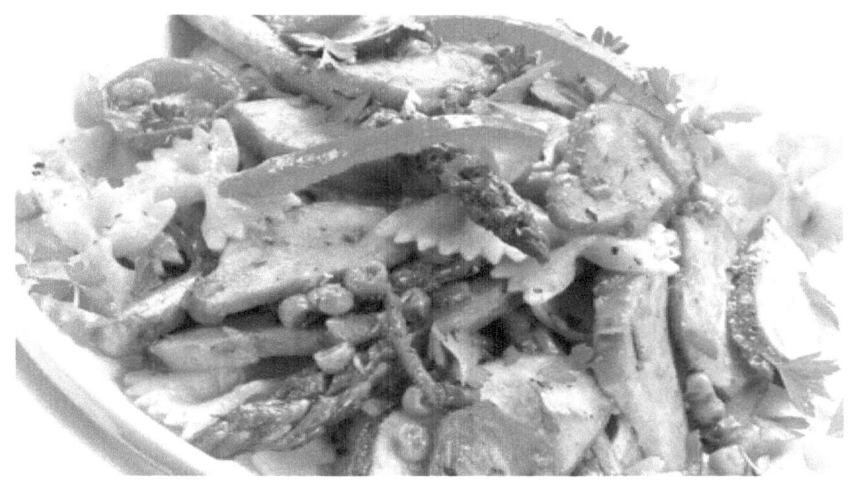

(1)   BOWTYE PASTA SUPPER SALAD

(2)

So whether you eat or drink or whatever you do, do it all for the glory of God.

[1 Corinthians 10:3]

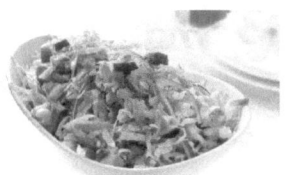

(2) PINK LADY COLD SLAW SUPPER SALAD

Ingredients

* 1 small cabbage head

* 2 large carrots grated

* 1/3 cup of red sweet onions

* 3 celery stalks diced

* 1 cup cubed zucchini

* 1 cup of pink lady apples, cubed

COLD SLAW DRESSING

Ingredients

* 1 cup olive oil, cracked pepper mayo

* 2 tbsp. brown vinegar

* 2 tbsp. light brown

* 1/2 tsp. dry mustard

* 1/4 tsp. paprika

 * 1/2 tsp. sea salt

Instructions

Mix dressing ingredients together in a bowl then pour over slaw salad toss together. Add favorite croutons or whole grain crackers for a tasty lunch or light supper.

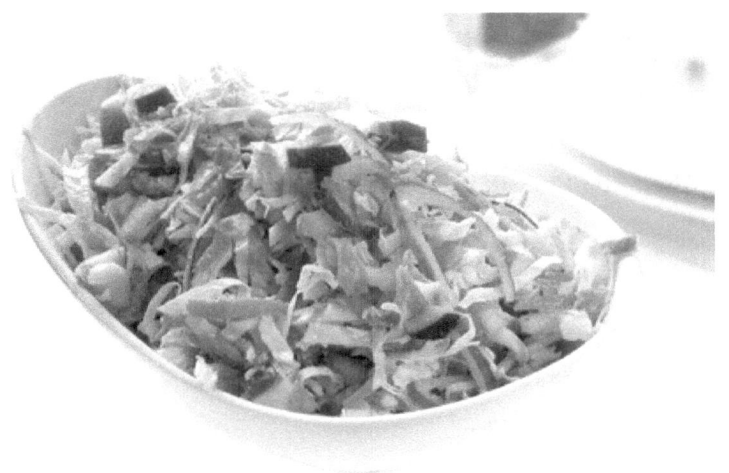

(3)   PINK LADY COLD SLAW SUPPER SALAD

Give thanks to the Lord, for He is good; His love endures forever.

[I Chronicles 16:34]

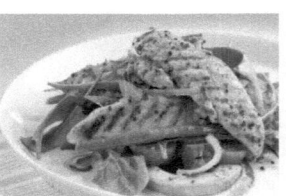

(4) WARM GRILLED CHICKEN SEASONED SALAD

Ingredients

4 pieces of raw chicken strips

1/4 cup of sautéed long fresh string green beans

2 cups of mixed salad greens, with spinach

1 large tomato - sliced

1 large avocado - sliced

1/3 cup thinly sliced red sweet onions

1 tsp grilled chicken seasoning mix

Directions

Season raw chicken strips to taste. Grill, and then set aside.   Add to eating dish your baby spinach, salad greens, plus sliced avocado, red sweet onions, fried green beans. Add a little balsamic low-fat dressing of choice or eat as is. Yummy pleasure! Very fulfilling!

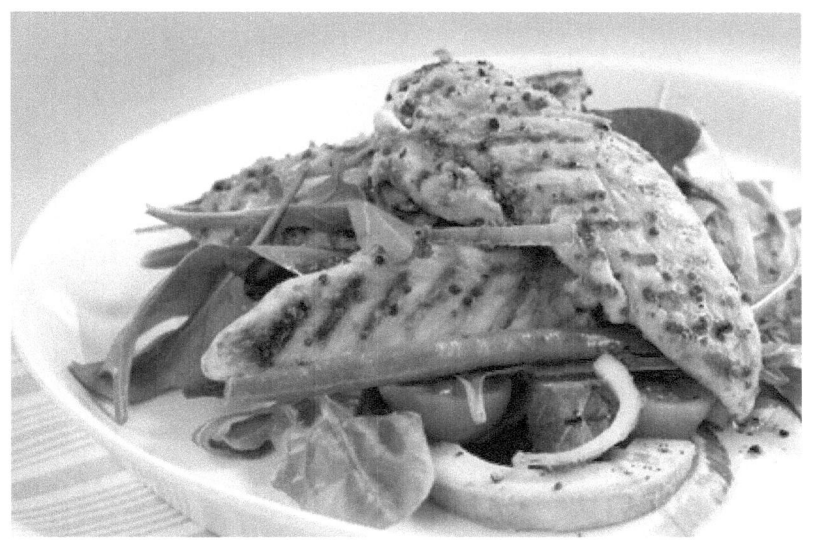

(3) WARM GRILLED SEASONED CHICKEN SUPPER SALAD

Give thanks to the Lord, call on His name; make known among the nations what he has done.

[I Chronicles 16:8]

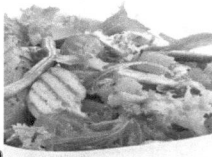

(4) BIT OF MEAT –N- VEGGIE SUPPER SALAD

This salad can be topped with any kind of white meat, i.e., - White Turkey, White Chicken, White Tuna or White Meat pork.

Ingredients

2 cups of organic salad greens (best choice)

1/2 cup fresh green beans

1/4 cup cubed bells, red, and yellow

1/4 cup of baby grape tomatoes

1/4 cup diced white meat, of choice...

Toss together in a bowl and serve with...

 * Fat free oil dressing of choice

Extra Flavor Bonus: add a hint of supper salad topping choices:

* Cracked pepper

* Sea salt

* Croutons

*Sun flower seeds

* Slivered almonds

*Pumpkin seeds

*Fennel

*Parsley

*Dill

*Coriander

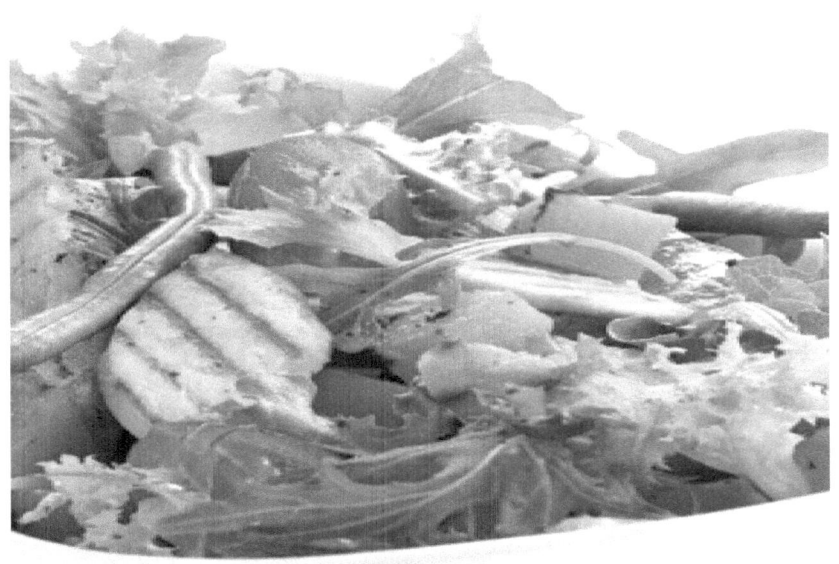

(5)   A BIT OF MEAT

VEGGIE SUPPER SALAD

The Lord is my strength and my shield; my heart trusts in Him, and I am helped.

[Psalm 28:7a]

(6) SMART EXPRESS SPAGETTI - LUNCH OR SUPPER

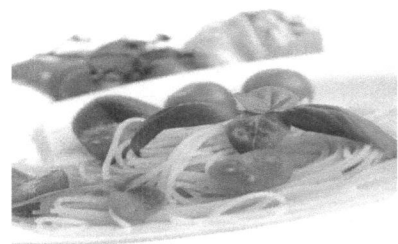

Ingredients

*2 cups of medium size spaghetti

*1 cup of mini – grape tomatoes

*1 tsp of virgin olive oil –

*1 tbsp of dried organic oregano seasoning

*1/3 cup of Romano cheese on top

*A pinch of all natural chili & dill sea salt to taste

Directions

Bring spaghetti to boil in pot of water, and then drain water off spaghetti when done. Set aside and warm up wok skillet putting in a cap of olive oil. Throw pasta spaghetti into warm skillet then mix in seasoning ingredients…Oregano - Chili dill sea salt. Stir together, then remove from heat and add to salad plate top with tomatoes and cheeses.

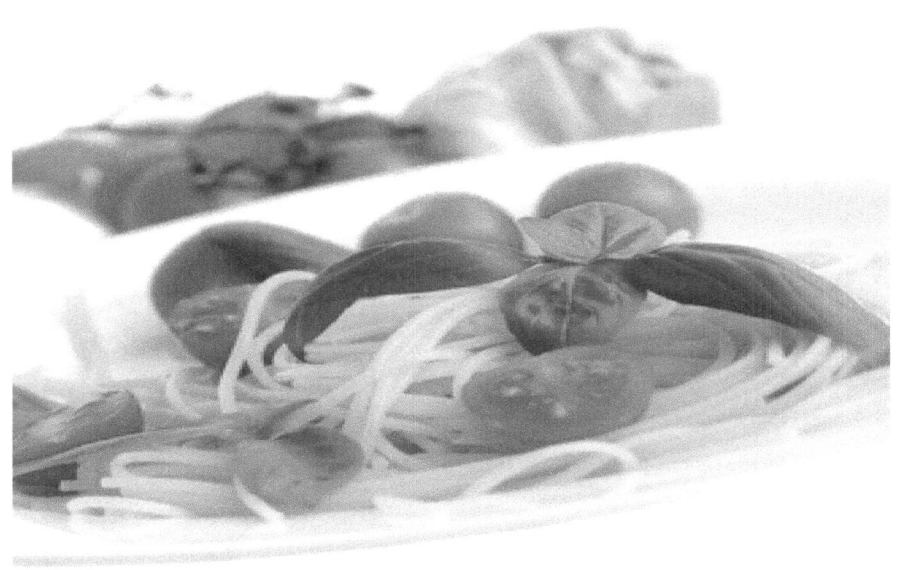

(5) SMART EXPRESS SPAGETTI - LUNCH OR SUPPER

Enter into His gates with thanksgiving, and into His courts with praise; be thankful unto Him, and bless His name. [Psalm100]

(6) PURPLE COLORED SIMPLE SALAD

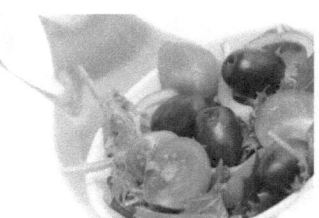

Ingredients

* 4 cups of organic greens

*1/4 cup of Purple Olives

*1/4 cup of Purple Onions

*1/4 cup of Grape Tomatoes

*1/3 cup of Wine Grapes (optional)

*1/4 cup of dried cranberries (optional)

*1 tbsp of Purple Creamy Balsamic Dressing

*A pinch of ground black pepper, savor & enjoy.

Directions

TOSS: together in a beautiful salad bowl all ingredients. Drizzle with dressings, then add pinch of lemon pepper and seas salt stir and enjoy.

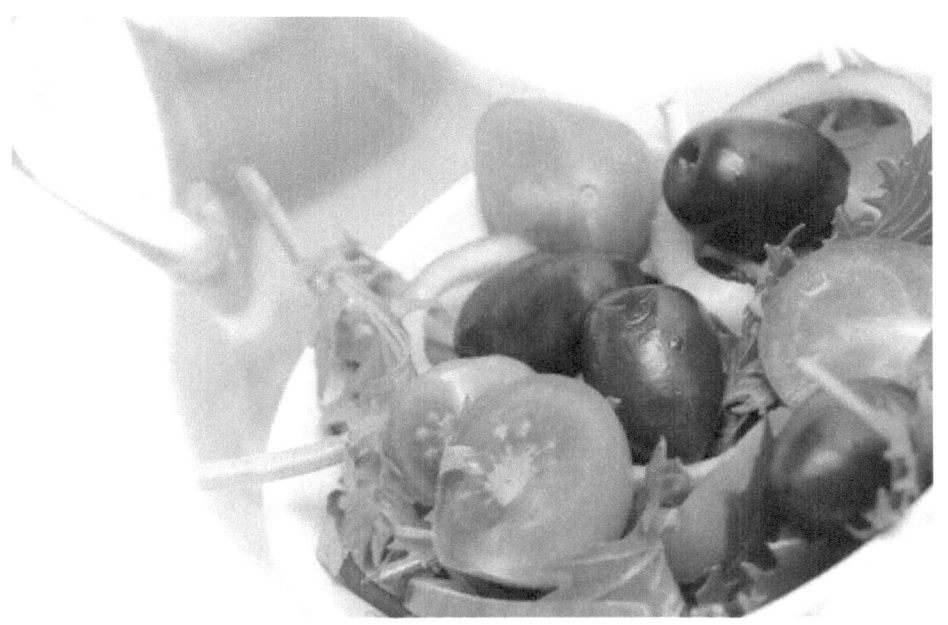

(7)   PURPLE COLORED SIMPLE SALAD

Better to have a dish of vegetables where there is love than juicy steaks where there is hate.

[Proverbs 15:7]

Have as your supper dessert or serve as a Lunch Treat –

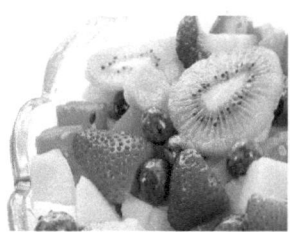

(7) HEALTHY FRESH FRUIT SALAD –

Ingredients

  *¼ cup Kiwi

  *¼ cup Pineapple

  * ¼ cup Watermelon

  *¼ cup Peach

  *¼ cup Blueberries

  *¼ cup Blackberries

  *¼ cup Honeydew

  *¼ cup Strawberries

Directions

Dice individual fruit, and then measure each to ¼ cup full. Mixing together in salad bowl and serve with...

Add any of the following fruit dressings:

- Strawberry balsamic dressing
- Orange cranberry dressing
- Peach pecan dressing
- Or Light raspberry dressing

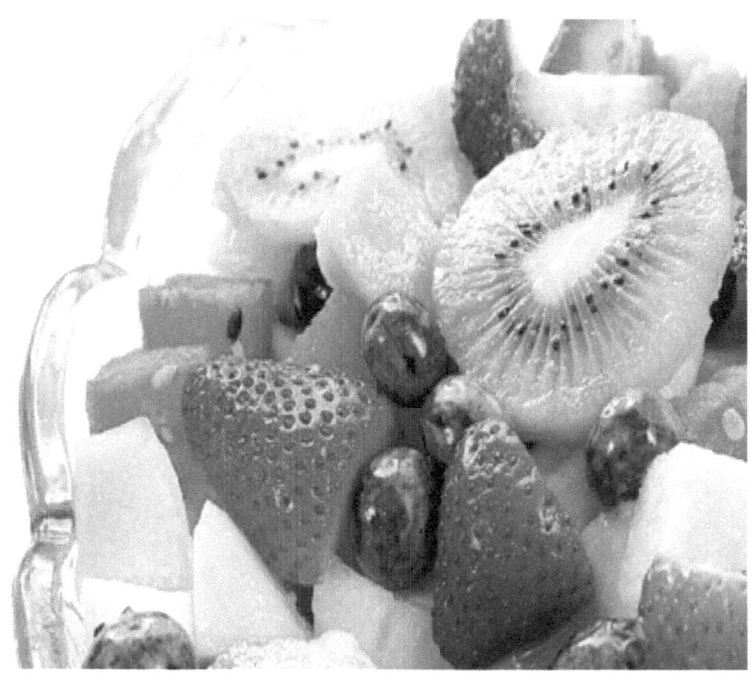

(8)   HEALTHY FRESH EXPRESS FRUIT SALAD

And the fruit of the Spirit is: Love, joy, peace, long-suffering, kindness, goodness, faith, meekness, and temperance: against such there is no law; [Galatians 5:22-23]

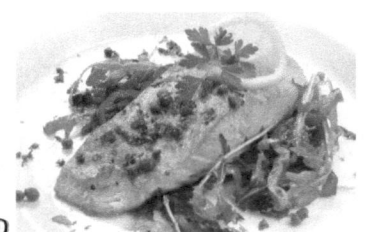

(9) SALMON SUPPER SALAD

Ingredients

*4 (6-ounce) salmon fillet

*1/2 cup olive oil

*1/2 teaspoon salt

*1/2 teaspoon pepper

*1/2 pound baby salad greens

*1 cup baby kalamata olives

*1peeled lemon slice

*1 small red bell pepper, thinly sliced

Directions

Preheat grill to hot, then place the salmon fillets on a large plate and coat with 1/4 cup real butter or olive oil, 1/4 teaspoon natural sea salt, and 1/4 teaspoon lemon or plain pepper. Put the salmon fillet on hot grill, skinless side down first. Cook for 5 to 10 minutes on each side, or until desired doneness.

While the salmon is grilling, combine the salad greens, olives, bell peppers and seasonings in a large bowl with your favorite vinaigrette dressing. When salmon is done remove from the grill lay on favorite supper plate for extra appealing mouth watering food venture. Place salmon on top of the salad greens mixture, and drizzle more dressing over salmon. Say your grace and eat up!

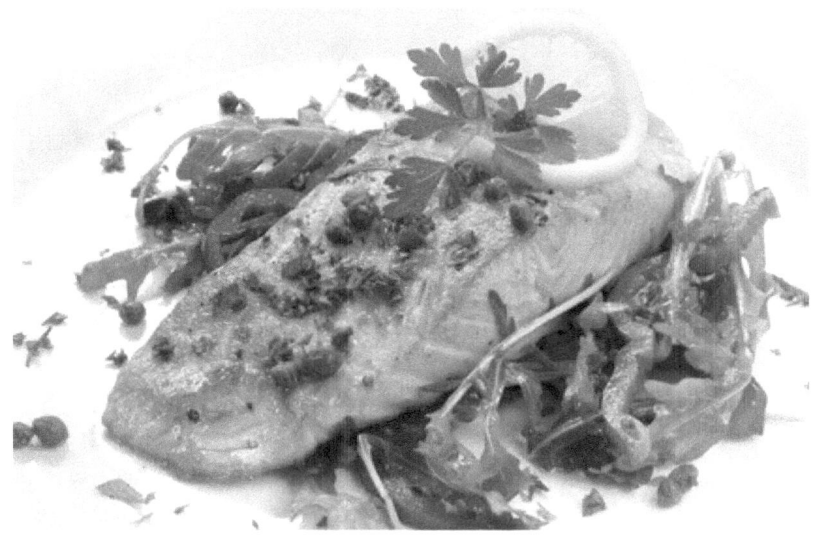

(8) SALMON SUPPER SALAD

Taking the five loaves and the two fish and looking up to heaven, he gave thanks and broke them. Then he gave them to the disciples to set before the people.

[Like 9:16]

(9) FETTUCINE CARBONARO PULLED PORK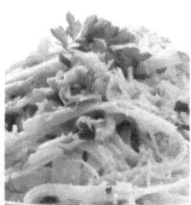

Ingredients

*3 tsp olive oil

*1small onion, cut into thin strips

*1 pound pulled pork, cooked/set aside

*1 garlic, clove chopped

*1 (16 ounce) package fettuccini pasta

*3/4 cup shredded Parmesan cheese

*Add salt and pepper to taste, herbs: green sprig of parsnip

Directions

Heat olive oil in a large heavy saucepan over medium heat - sauté onion and cooked pork together, stirring in garlic when pork is browned a little. Remove to cool burner. Bring a large pot of lightly salted water with a cap full of olive oil to a boil. Add pasta and cook for 8 to 10 minutes or until done. Drain pasta, and move to a medium bowl. Then add meat and seasonings mixture to top of pasta, put on supper plates and sprinkle with some shredded Parmesan or Ramona cheese, then season a little more with salt and pepper, a green sprig of parsnip. Bring to the table as a mouth watering delectable piece. Delicious!

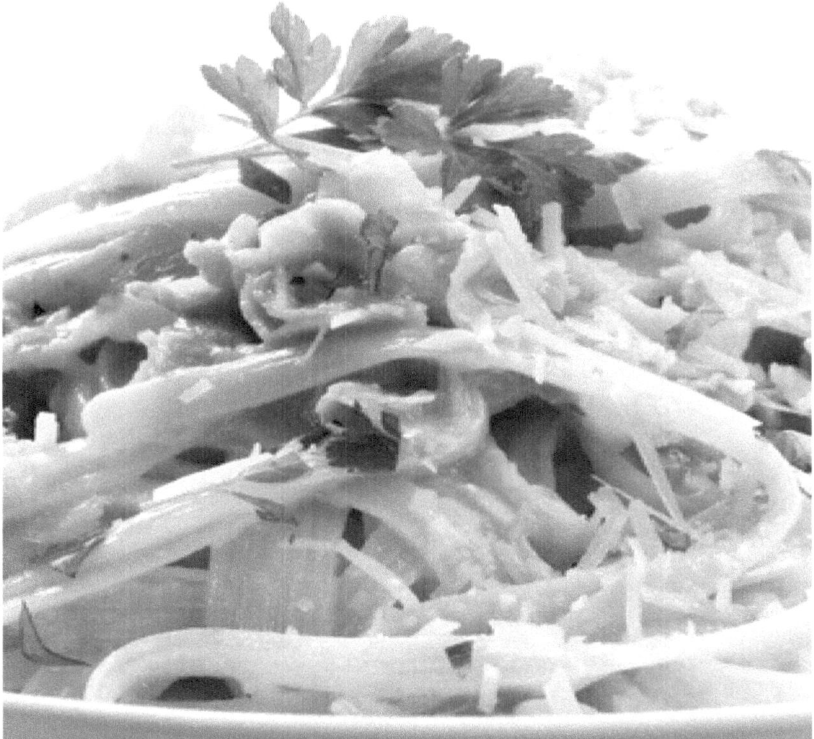

(9) FETTUCINE CARBONARA PULLED PORK SUPPER

Try

While dining with a ruler, pay attention to what is put before you.

[Proverbs 23:1]

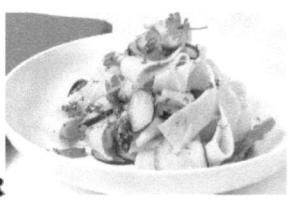

(10)PAPPARDELLE COURGETTE SUPPER

Ingredients

* 1 tbsp butter

* 1 tbsp sunflower oil

*1-1/2 or (4 medium) courgettes

*1 clove garlic, minced

*Sea salt, dill chili sea pepper

*2-3 tbsp Marsala (wine)

*4-6 long stemmed asparagus

1/2 cup of chopped tomatoes

8 oz egg pappardelle noodles

4 tbsp freshly grated Parmesan

Small bunch fresh parsley, chopped

Directions:

Wash the courgette in cold water cut off the top and tail and throw away. Cut into slices about 5 mm wide. Heat the butter and sunflower oil in a saucepan, and put the cut courgettes (or substitute zucchini) into hot saucepan. Mince in the garlic and season with sea salt and dill chili sea pepper. Cook over medium heat for about 25 minutes, stirring occasionally. Then add asparagus stems cooking for 15 minutes more. When ready the courgettes or zucchini will have sweated down. (The salt draws the moisture out, making firm for salad) Next, pour in chopped tomatoes and simmer on low for 5 minutes more. Meanwhile, warm the Marsala (wine), pour over the cooked courgettes/zucchini/asparagus and tomatoes mixture. Then stir in juices, to season taste a bit more. Cook pasta according to pkg instructions, drain, and tip into warmed bowl. Add courgette mixture, fold and toss to combine. Sprinkle parmesan and most of chopped parsley and toss everything together gently. Serve for a scrumptious supper meal or smart tasty lunch.

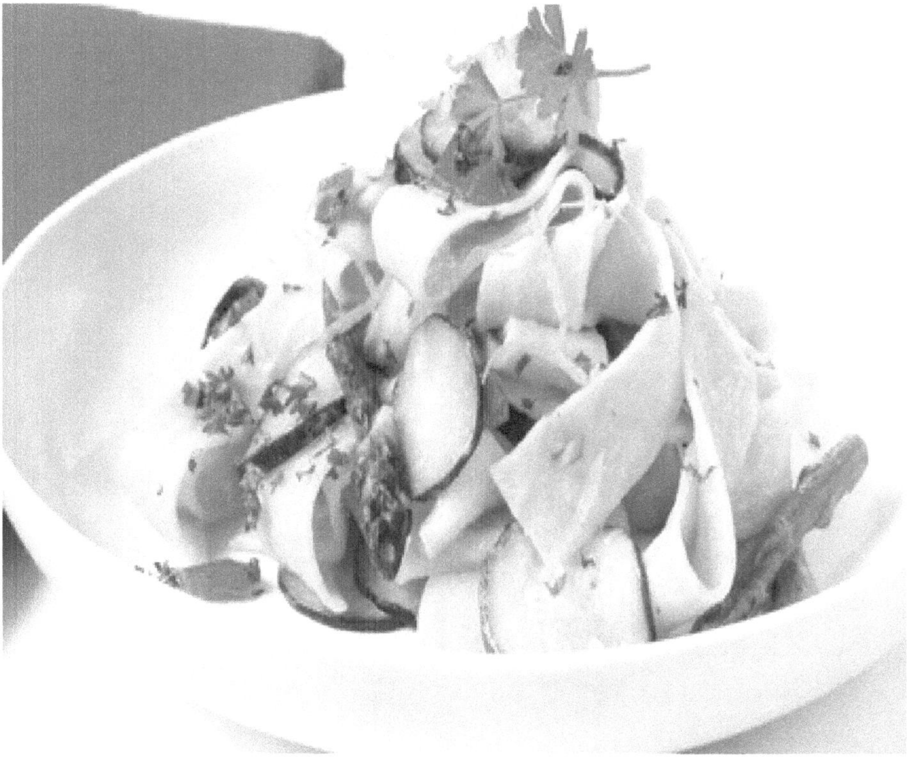

(10) PAPPARDELLE COURGETTE SUPPER

Try

And God said, "Behold, I have given you every plant yielding seed that is on the face of all the earth, and every tree with seed in its fruit. You shall have them for food.[Genesis 1:29]

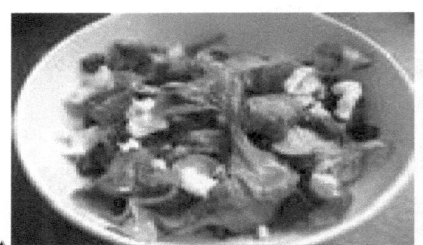

(11) SIMPLE SPINACH BEETS BOWL

Ingredients

*One 10-12 oz can of red sliced beets or

*2 tablespoon(s) red wine vinegar

*1 teaspoon(s) Dijon mustard

*1/4 cup(s) olive oil

*1 1/2 teaspoon(s) sugar

*1/8 teaspoon(s) salt

*Dash of pepper to season

*1/2 cup(s) chopped green onion stems

*1/2 teaspoon(s) minced fresh mint

*4 cup(s) torn fresh spinach

*1/2 cup(s) fresh raspberries

* 1 / 2 cup of feta cheese

** Optional (Dash of chili powder)

Directions

In a small bowl stir vinegar and mustard until blended; gradually whisk in oil. Add sugar, salt and pepper, chili powder and combine the beets, onions, mint and 2 tablespoons vinaigrette. Cover and refrigerate for 20 minutes. In a large salad bowl, combine the spinach, beet mixture and remaining vinaigrette; toss. Top with raspberries and feta cheese. Serve immediately.

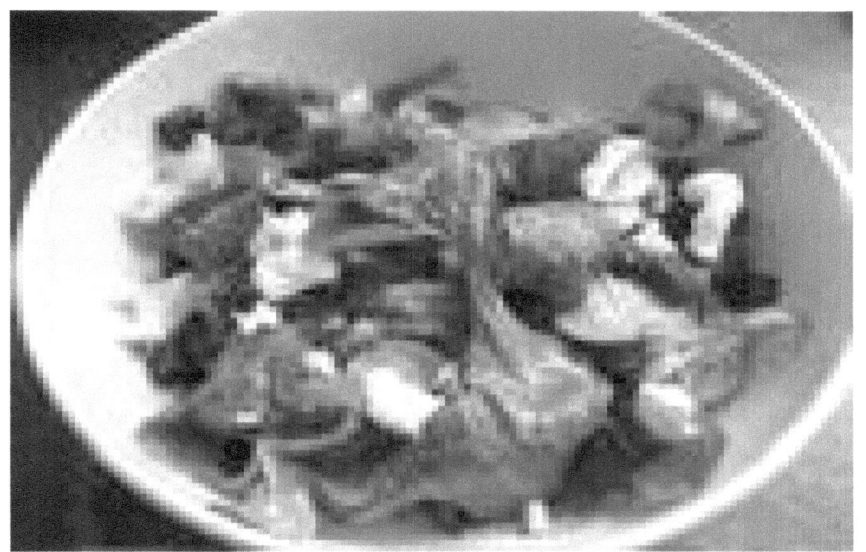

(11) SIMPLE SPINACH BEETS BOWL LUNCH

Every moving thing that lives shall be food for you. And as I gave you the green plants, I give you everything. [Genesis 9:3]

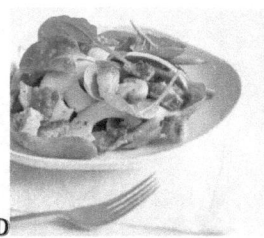

(12)YUM BABY – BACON BISTRO SPINACH SALAD

Ingredients

* 4-6 strips of bacon

*1-2 large avocados

*1 cup fresh mushrooms

*1 can of garbanzo beans

*4 cups baby leaf spinach

*1/2 cups of bread croutons

* Bacon oil/grease

**pinch of salt, pepper and dry Ramona cheese powder

Directions

Fry the bacon till crisp, drain grease and set aside. Drop bread croutons into bacon fat and brown with salt and pepper seasoning. Set aside to cool. Tip sliced mushrooms into bacon fat to rid of rawness a bit then when cooled add to salad bowl. Open can of beans toss into salad bow along with sliced avocado, then lastly add baby spinach to mixture, crumble bacon into bowl, drizzling over with your favorite dressing, and dry Ramona cheese, coating well. Eat till your tummy's overjoyed.

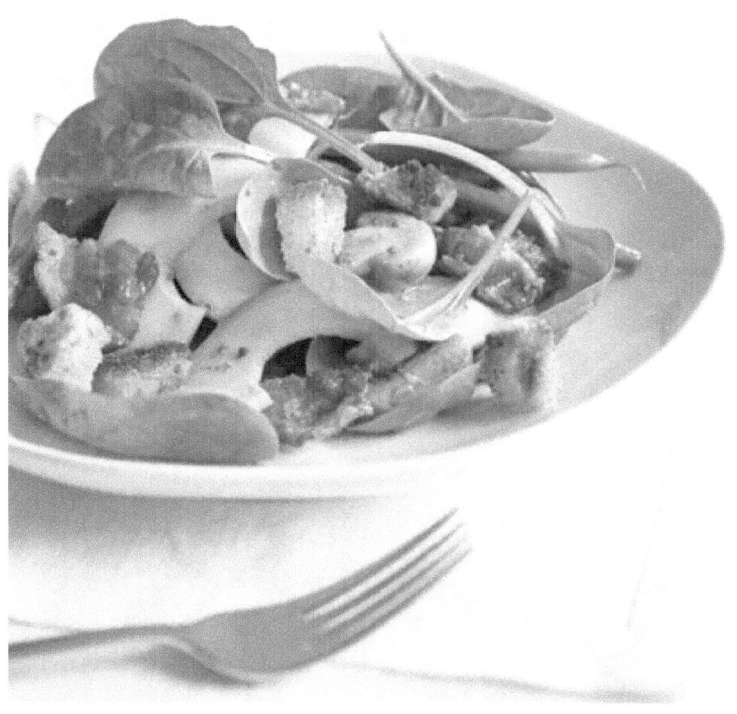

(12)YUM BABY – BACON BISTRO SPINACH SALAD

I am the Lord your God, who brought you up out of the land of Egypt. Open your mouth wide, and I will fill it. [Psalms 81:10]

(13) CHICKEN RICOTTA SALAD

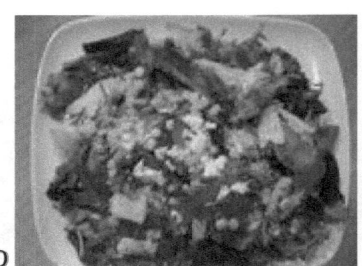

Ingredients

1 small bag of Spinach leaves

425 grams of low fat ricotta

One 10-12 oz can of four bean mix

One 10-12 oz can of corn kernels

Half a red onion thinly sliced

1 large can of white meat chunky chicken

Low- fat balsamic vinegar dressing

Directions

Rinse spinach leaves and spread evenly at the bottom salad bowl, then in a separate bowl mix corn, ricotta chicken and beans till ricotta is distributed evenly. Spread this mix over the spinach leaves. Chill in fridge for 15-20 minutes. After the drizzle of dressing over mix, quickly serve, to enjoy.

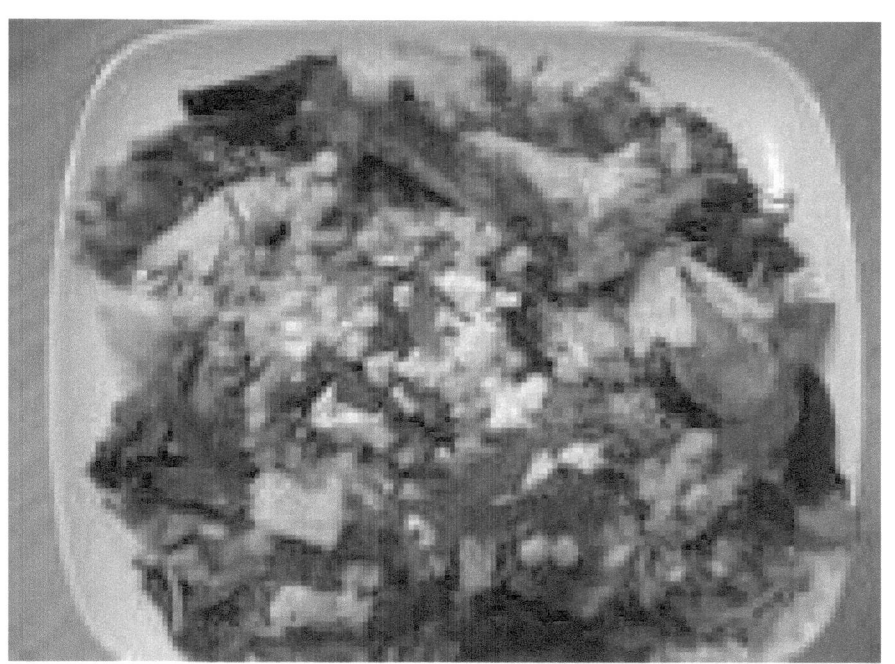

(13) CHICKEN RICOTTA SALAD

But I discipline my body and keep it under control, lest after preaching to others I myself should be disqualified. [1 Corinthians 9:27]

(14) CHICKEN ROTINI BROCCOLI CASSEROLE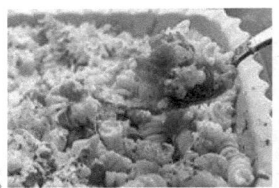

Ingredients:

*4-6 pieces boneless skinless chicken breast, cooked, square diced

*8 ounces rotini pasta, cooked as directed on pkg, drained

*1 tablespoon olive oil

*1/2 cup chopped onion

*2 cloves garlic, finely minced

*1 can (14.5 ounces) diced tomatoes, undrained

* 2 large broccoli florets

*1/2 teaspoon dried leaf basil

*Dash chili pepper

*Dash of white pepper

*Dash of black pepper

*1/2 teaspoon sea salt

*1 1/2 cups shredded Mexican cheese, divided

Directions

Grease a 2-quart baking dish or spray with nonstick cooking spray-Heat oven to 350° Heat oil in a medium saucepan and brown cubed chicken breast add onion and sauté for about 3 to 5 minutes, until onion is tender. Add the garlic, tomatoes, and basil; cook for 2 minutes more, until heated through. Taste and add the white pepper, sea salt, chili pepper, making adjustments to suit your taste. In another small pot, boil rotini and broccoli till tender then drain and Stir into chicken mix. Stir in 1 cup of the cheese; spoon into the prepared baking dish. Sprinkle remaining shredded cheese over the top of the casserole. Bake for 20 to 25 minutes, until hot and bubbly. Serves 6 med. - supper plates! Mmm – Good!

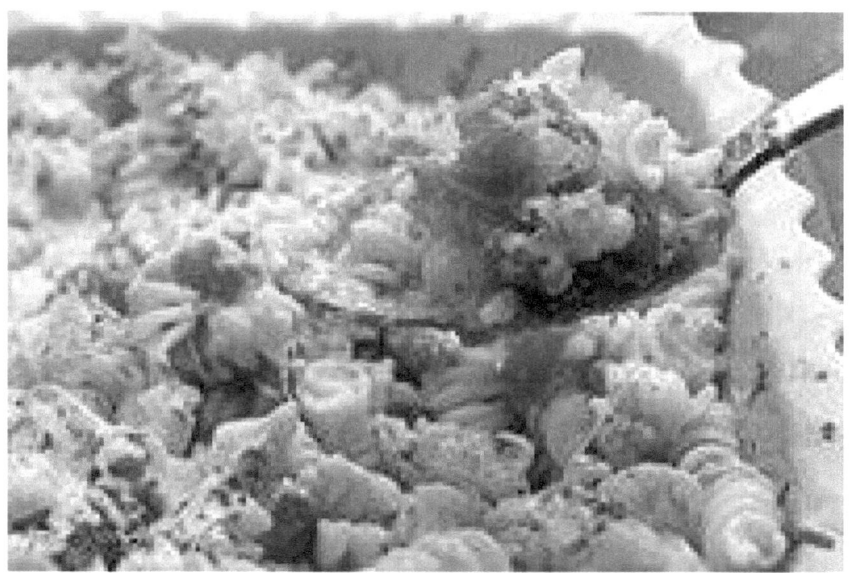

(14) CHICKEN ROTINI BROCCOLI CASSEROLE

Jesus said to them, "I am the bread of life; whoever comes to me shall not hunger, and whoever believes in me shall never thirst. [John 6:35]

(15) COBB SALAD

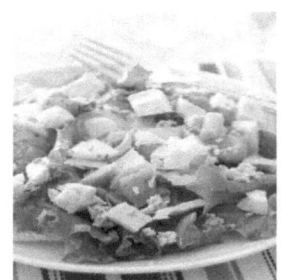

Ingredients

* 1 1/2 cups of white meat chicken

*1/4 teaspoon sea salt

*1/4 teaspoon ground black pepper

*6 cups mixed greens

*1 cup diced or halved tomatoes, (any kind)

*2 tablespoons sliced green onion stems

*fat-free Italian dressing to suit taste

*1 ½ tablespoons crumbled blue cheese

*1- 2 crumbled boiled eggs

Directions

Combine greens, tomatoes, onion stems, in a large bowl. Drizzle greens mixture with dressing, then add sea salt and ground pepper, tossing gently to coat. Arrange salad mixture on salad plate, tip on top, separately the chicken, then layer with crumbled eggs and crumbled blue cheese and serve.   Simple and delectable!

Add whole grain crackers on the side, to this supper salad.

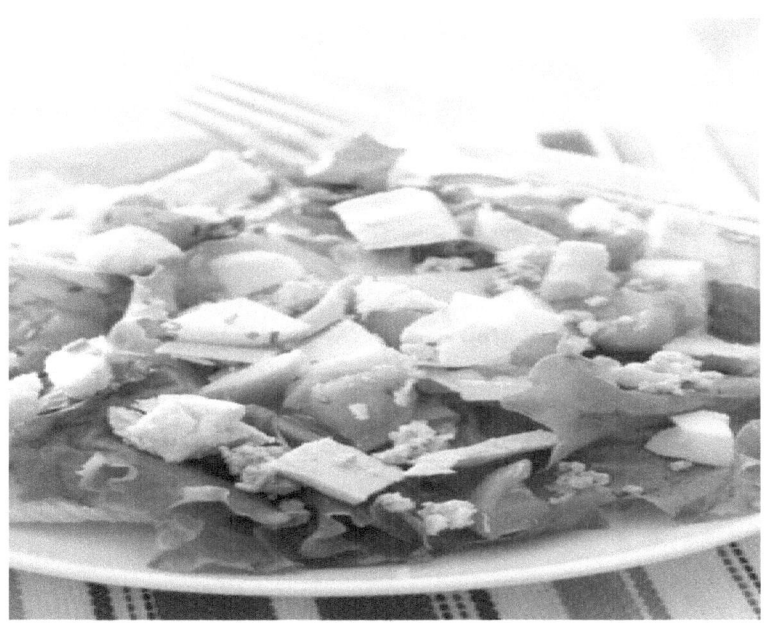

(15) COBB SALAD

I appeal to you therefore, brothers, by the mercies of God, to present your bodies as a living sacrifice, holy and acceptable to God, which is your spiritual worship. [Romans 12:1]

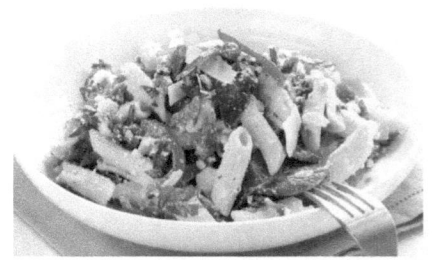

(16) COLD SPINACH ROTINI PASTA SALAD

Ingredients

* 8 oz Penne Pasta

* 3 cups torn spinach

* 1 medium Red Bell Pepper, thinly sliced

* 12 cherry tomatoes, sliced in half

* 1/2 cup Italian type salad dressing

* 1 cup of shredded Gouda-cheese

* A pinch of salt, chili powder, turmeric & pepper

* 3 tablespoons of mozzarella cheese

Directions

Toss all raw vegetables, including tomatoes, into large salad bowl, pour on partial dressing to   mix thoroughly with seasonings. Set aside in fridge while pasta is cooking. When pasta is done, drain and rinse with cold water, let cool for 10 minutes. Then add pasta and cheese to vegetable mixture - layer on plates, drizzle more dressing of choice to taste satisfaction.

Add a little protein to your Penne by adding: any of the meat/nut choices:
 * Chicken breast, *white meat tuna, *salmon or *toasted pine nuts or raw walnuts

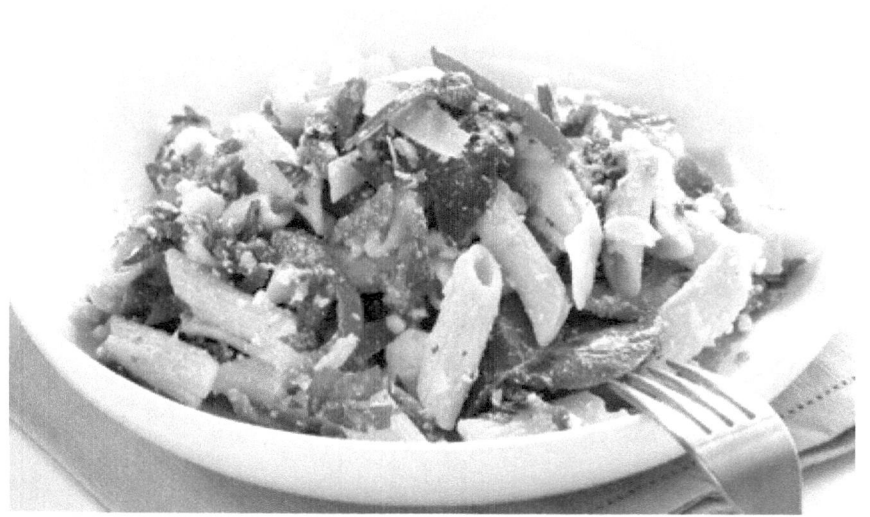

(16) COLD SPINACH ROTINI PASTA SALAD

Blessed shall be your basket and your kneading bowl.

[Deuteronomy 28:5]

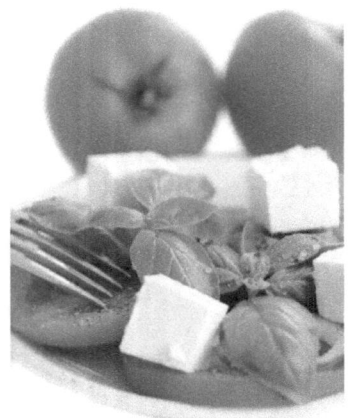

(17) FETA & TOMATO APPETIZER SALAD

Ingredients

Your ingredients will vary with this tasty simplistic appetizer, according to how many guest.

* 3-6 large organic red tomatoes, sliced

*A dozen fresh basil leaves

*1 carton of feta cheese

*Sea salt chili dill seasoning to taste

*1/2 cup balsamic vinegar

*1/4 cup extra virgin olive oil

Directions

Be creative with decorating- Place sliced tomatoes on bottom of server, sprinkle with seasoning salts, peppers. Layer on top the cheese squares with fresh basil intertwined between the two. Mix the vinegar and oil together in a small bowl to serve. Allowing guest to add or eat alone.

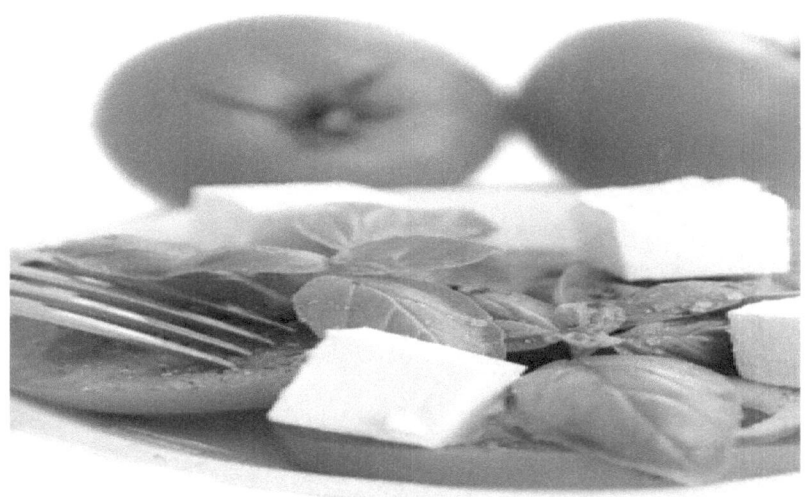

(17) FETA & TOMATO APPETIZER SALAD

The humble will inherit the land, and will delight themselves in abundant prosperity

[Psalm 37:11]

GREEN RIBBON FETTUCINE CARBONARO

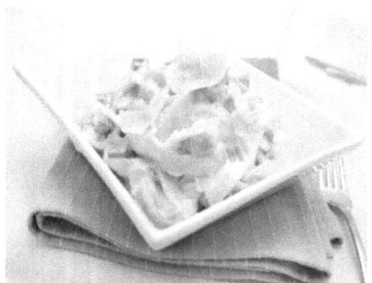

(18) LACED WITH BACON & TURKEY

Ingredients

*375g dried green and white fettuccine pasta

*½ pack 98% fat free bacon, cut into 1.5cm pieces

*2 large cans white breast turkey meat

*1 Jar of white creamy fettuccine sauce

*1/3 cup, lightly packed coarsely grated reduced-fat cheddar

* Desired amount of shaved parmesan, to serve

Directions

Cook pasta in a saucepan of boiling water following packet directions or until texture desired. Drain and set aside. Meanwhile, heat a non-stick frying pan over medium-high heat. Add bacon and cook for 5 minutes or until crisp, then transfer to a plate. Heat the creamy sauce in a saucepan over medium heat. Add the cheddar and parmesan and stir until melted. Add the pasta mixture, cans of turkey and tender bacon mixture to the pan and stir until combined. Divide among serving bowls. Season with salt and pepper and top with more shaved parmesan. Serve with pleasure.

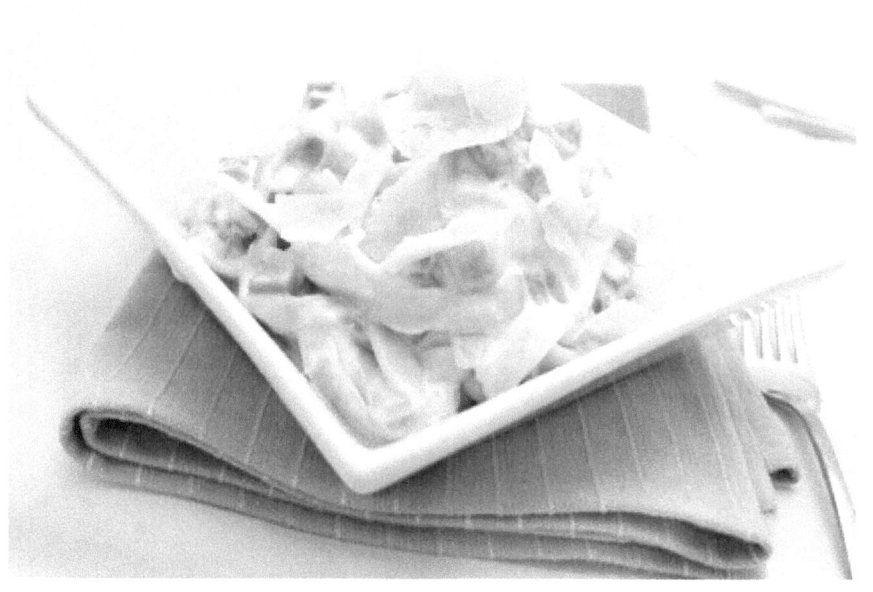

(18) GREEN RIBBON FETTUCINE CARBONARO

LACED WITH BACON & TURKEY

And put a knife to your throat if you are given to gluttony (appetite)

[Proverbs 23:2]

(19) SMART & EASY TOSSED SUPPER SALAD

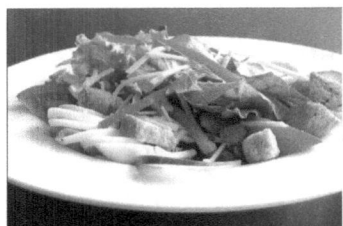

This easy breezy tossed green salad can be thrown together in a jiffy!

Ingredients:

*1 small head romaine or leaf lettuce, or enough salad greens for 2-4 people

*2 green onions sliced or (substitute with sweet red onion slices)

*1/2 to 1 cucumber sliced

*1 red, orange or yellow bell pepper, thinly sliced

*4 hard boiled eggs

*Organic tomatoes, wedged

*Mild cheddar cheese grated

* Croutons of choice

* Herbs: vary with taste buds

- 1 cup fresh coriander /cilantro, roughly chopped
- 1/2 cup fresh basil, roughly chopped
- Salad dressing: (double recipe if serving 4 or more)
- 1 Tbsp. lime juice

Directions:

Prep all veggie greens in large salad bowl, mix in herbs of choice and then lay out on salad/ supper plate evenly. Squeeze lime juice over greens. Add tomato wedges, sliced eggs on the side and salt, pepper and salad dressing. Top off with croutons and grated cheese.

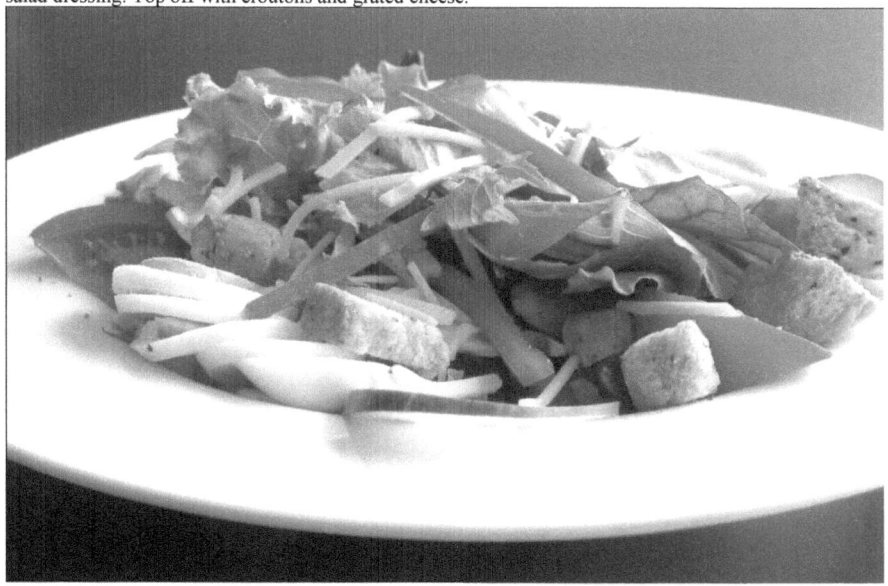

(19) SMART & EASY TOSSED SUPPER SALAD

So let each one give as he purposes in his heart, not grudgingly, or of necessity: for God loves a cheerful giver. [2 Corinthians 9:7b]

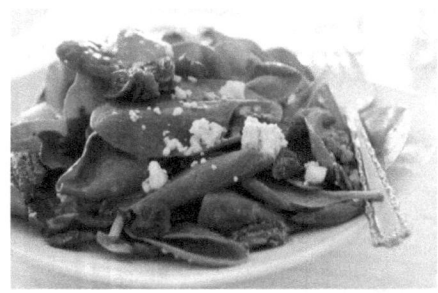

(20) POPEYE SPINACH SALAD

Ingredients

*4-6 cups of organic spinach

*2 tablespoons of blue cheese

*1 cup of dried red cranberries

*½ cup of walnuts or pecans

*Favorite dressing of choice

Simple, healthy and very - very good!

Directions:

Not a problem! Just open a bag of delicious organic baby spinach Add dried fruit (cranberries) nuts and cheese, drizzle dressing sauce and eat till full.

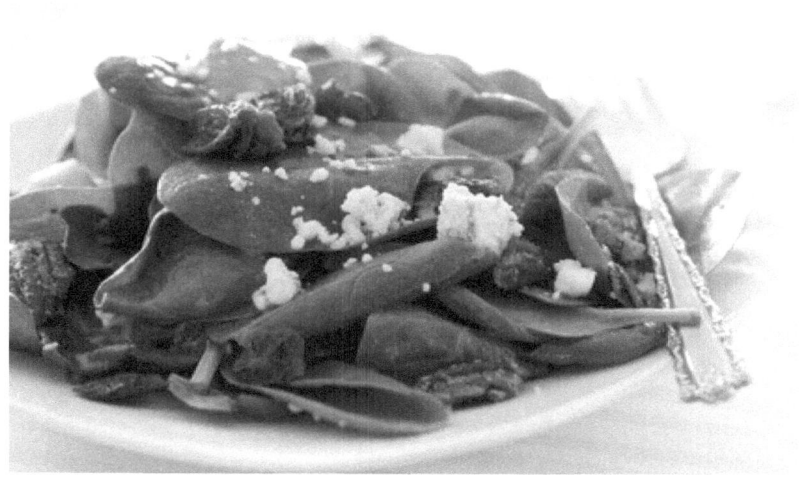

SPINACH SALAD

"And you, take wheat and barley, beans and lentils, millet and emmer, and put them into a single vessel and make your bread from them. During the number of days that you lie on your side, 390 days, you shall eat it. [Ezekiel 4:9]

www.ingramcontent.com/pod-product-compliance
Lightning Source LLC
Chambersburg PA
CBHW061231280526
45784CB00006B/2718